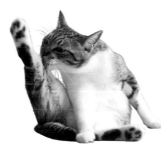

YOGA with CATS

31 Yoga Stretches Inspired by Cats

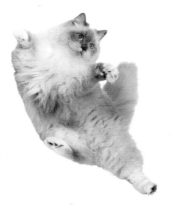

YOGA with CATS

Have you ever wondered if cats were true yoga masters?
The way they move and stretch, how they can be playful one
minute and totally relaxed the next—they are extraordinary to
watch! Motivated by the movements of our feline friends, we
created a book to show 31 simple, cat-inspired yoga stretches
and poses.

Yoga was developed thousands of years ago to calm the
mind through a physical and mental practice. But the physical
side of modern-day yoga can be a bit intimidating for people
who have never done it before or have tighter bodies. If you
dropped two balls from a second-story window and one was
glass and the other was rubber, the glass ball would shatter,
while the rubber ball would simply bounce away down the
street. Likewise, a tight body can be more susceptible to
injuries than a limber body.

That's why it's important to move and stretch the body. But
the benefits are not just physical, they are good for your mind
as well, as there are positive effects to stopping for a few
moments a day to do something good for yourself.

Start slowly, and pick one pose—*any pose!*—and try it. You will
be amazed at how you feel after you start copying your cat.

Contents:

★ – Super Easy   ★★ – Somewhat Easy   ★★★ – Not So Easy

⟨ Before You Begin... ⟩

1 Avoid these stretches if you have pain or injuries.

If you have any injuries or illnesses or are simply not feeling well, just rest and enjoy the pictures instead! If you are currently pregnant or not sure if you should try one or more of these stretches, always consult with your physician.

2 Go barefoot.

It is nice to do these stretches without your socks or shoes, so you can feel the tactile sensation of the mat or the floor. Spread and stretch your toes, too.

3 Wear something comfortable.

You don't need fancy yoga clothes or special leggings that perform magic tricks, but wear something that won't restrict your movements but is not so loose the fabric is in your way.

4 Use a mat or towel.

You don't have to, but if it's available use a yoga or stretching mat, a towel, a cushion, or a blanket to support your body. These props help make the stretches more comfortable for your body. If you are using a towel or blanket, be careful not to slip!

The green highlights on the human diagram show the target of each stretch.

5   Don't forget to breathe.

Sometimes, if the sensation of the stretch is intense, we forget to breathe. Keep breathing! It is not only important physically, but a slow and steady breath also starts to calm your mind.

6   Hold the pose for several breaths.

You will see the instruction to hold the pose for five breaths. It could be fewer or more than that. The important thing is to take your time. Don't be in a hurry to strike a pose and move on.

7   Do what feels right for your body.

The pictures are visual references. Your pose may not look like the ones the human or feline models are doing. That's okay! Do what you can without pushing yourself too hard.

8   Stretch any time of the day.

If you stretch in the morning, it helps you wake up, and if you stretch at night, it helps you get the kinks out before bed. You can even try some of these poses on a break at work or between classes. In other words, try them anytime you want!

* The writer and the publisher are not responsible for any injuries that occur during stretching. Take necessary precautions, and stretch at your own risk.

Banzai!
Arms Up!

Raise your arms up, and stretch the sides of your body.

☑ Shoulders

☑ Arms

☑ Sides of your body

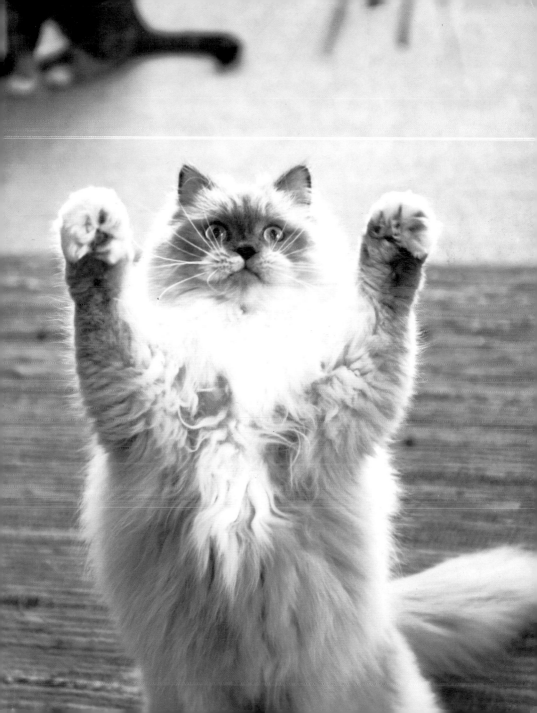

Banzai!
Arms Up!

Ground your feet firmly, and lift both arms overhead to stretch the sides of your body.

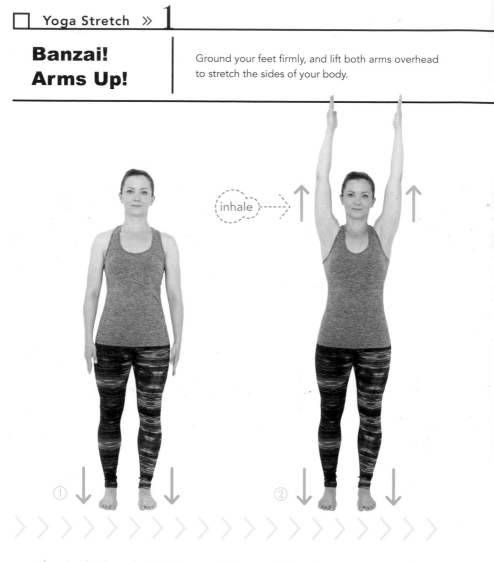

inhale ┈┈▶

1 Stand with your feet hip-width apart (AKA about two fists of space between your big toes). Think about rooting your feet down while lengthening your spine by reaching the top of your head toward the sky.

2 Lift your arms overhead as you inhale through your nose. Straighten your elbows even if you have to open your arms wider to do so.

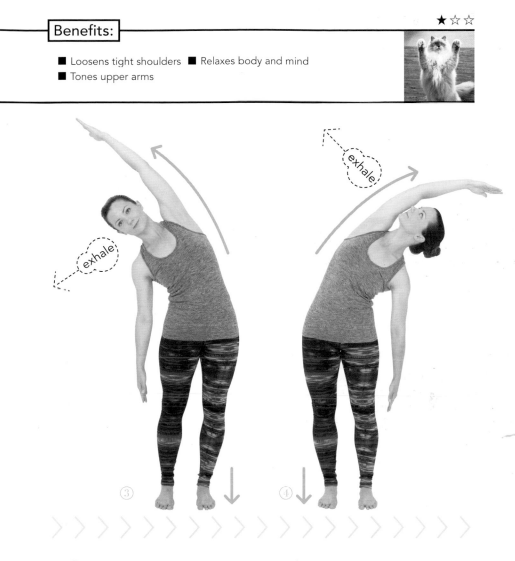

★ ☆ ☆

Benefits:

- Loosens tight shoulders ■ Relaxes body and mind
- Tones upper arms

exhale

exhale

③

④

> >

3 Lower your right arm by your side, and keep your left arm up. Side bend to the right as you exhale. Hold this stretch for five breaths.

4 Inhale to come back to the center, and exhale as you repeat these steps on the other side.

9

Forward Fold

Sit with your legs extended, and fold forward.

☑ Back

☑ Legs

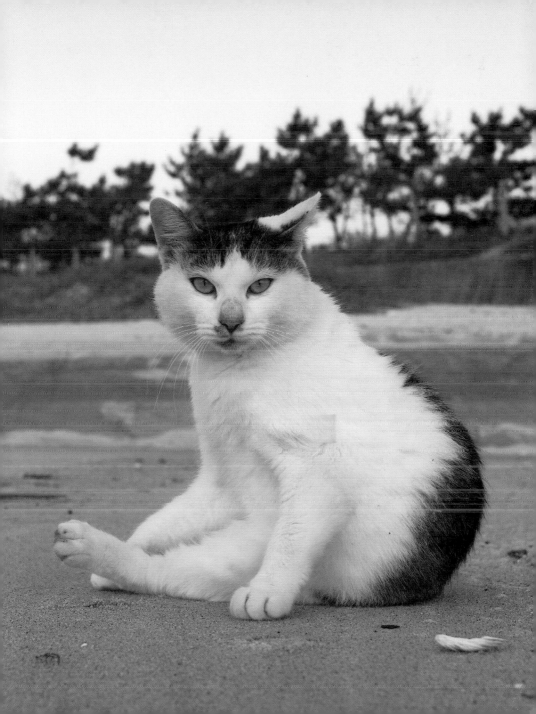

Forward Fold

From a seated position, lift your arms overhead, lengthen your spine, and fold forward into *paschimottanasana*, one of the most popular yoga poses.

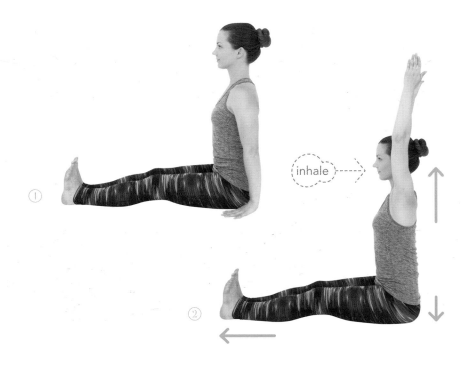

inhale

1. Sit with your legs extended in front of you, and lengthen your spine. If it's challenging to lengthen your spine, sit at the edge of a cushion or folded blanket to make it easier to stretch forward with a flat back, rather than stretching forward by rounding your back.

2. Raise your arms overhead to help lengthen the sides of your body as you inhale.

Benefits:

- Stretches the entire back of the body
- Helps improve digestion ■ Lessens fatigue
- May help alleviate headaches ■ Helps reduce stress

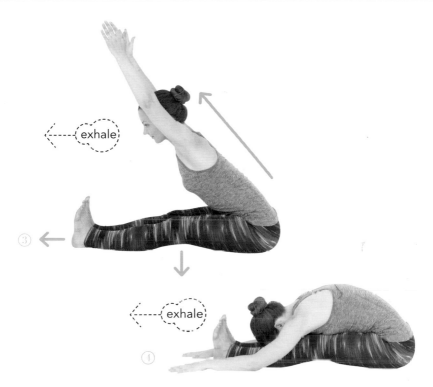

3 Hinging from your hips, fold forward as you exhale. Stop at the place where you feel a moderate stretch in your hamstrings, the big muscles at the back of each thigh. Stay for five breaths.

4 If it feels appropriate, fold a bit deeper, and hold for five more breaths.

13

Squat + Twist

Squat down, and twist around.

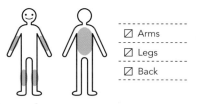

☑ Arms

☑ Legs

☑ Back

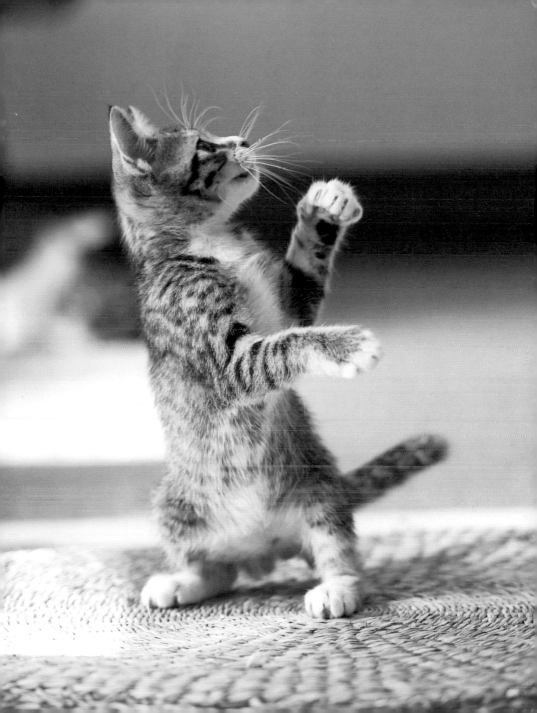

□ Yoga Stretch » 3

Squat + Twist

Squat down, bring your hands together in front of your heart, and gently twist to each side, optionally extending your arms, in this variation of *malasana*, or garland pose.

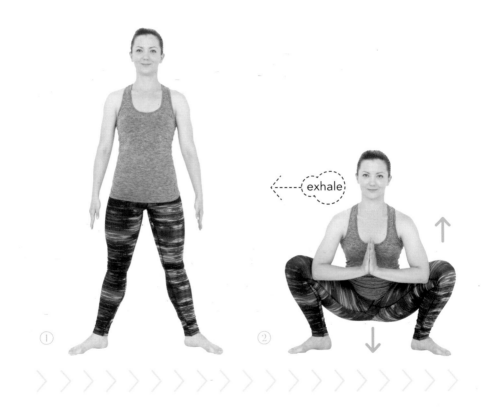

exhale

1. Stand with your feet wider than your hips with your toes turned out in the same direction as your knees.

2. Bring your hands together, and on an exhale, lower to a squat. Bring your elbows to your inner knees and press them against one another.

Benefits:

■ Strengthens legs ■ Helps reduce lower back pain
■ Improves flexibility in hip joints ■ Helps relieve constipation

exhale

exhale

③

①

> > > > > > > > > > > > > > > > > > > >

3 Extend your right arm in front of your right shin, bringing your hand or fingertips toward the floor. Extend your left arm diagonally away from your right arm, and start to twist to the left as you exhale. Hold for five breaths.

4 Bring yourself back to the center as you inhale, and repeat on the second side.

Tabletop to Plank

From a tabletop position,
extend your legs behind you into a plank pose.

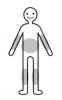

☑ Arms
☑ Abdomen
☑ Legs

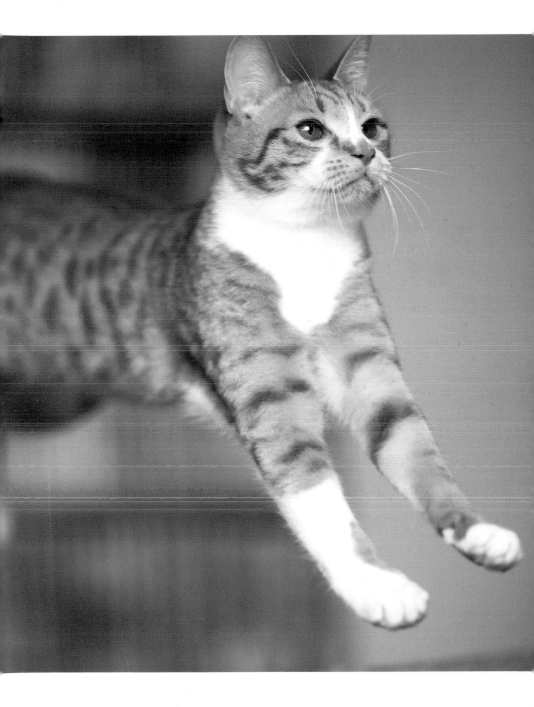

Tabletop to Plank

To try *kumbhakasana*, stretch your legs behind you, and come to a pushup preparation shape, staying strong and sturdy like a plank of wood.

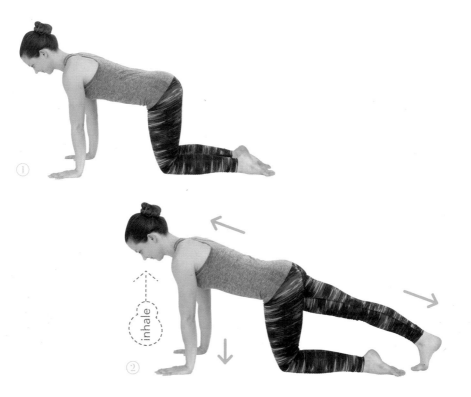

》 》 》 》 》 》 》 》 》 》 》 》 》 》 》 》 》

1 Come to all fours with your wrists directly under your shoulders and your knees directly under your hips.

2 Extend your right leg behind you on an inhale.

★ ★ ☆

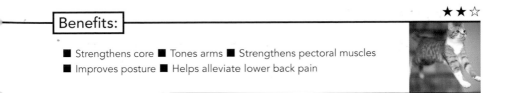

Benefits:

- ■ Strengthens core ■ Tones arms ■ Strengthens pectoral muscles
- ■ Improves posture ■ Helps alleviate lower back pain

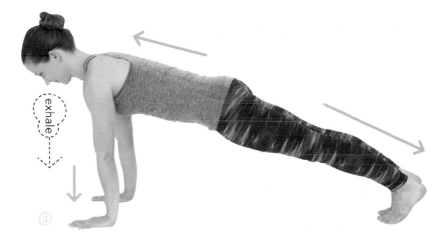

exhale

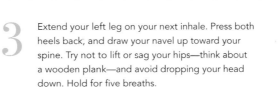

3 Extend your left leg on your next inhale. Press both heels back, and draw your navel up toward your spine. Try not to lift or sag your hips—think about a wooden plank—and avoid dropping your head down. Hold for five breaths.

21

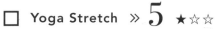

Reach Up in Triangle

With your legs wide, lean your torso forward,
and reach your hands wide from Earth to sky.

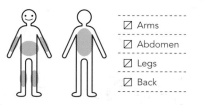

☑ Arms

☑ Abdomen

☑ Legs

☑ Back

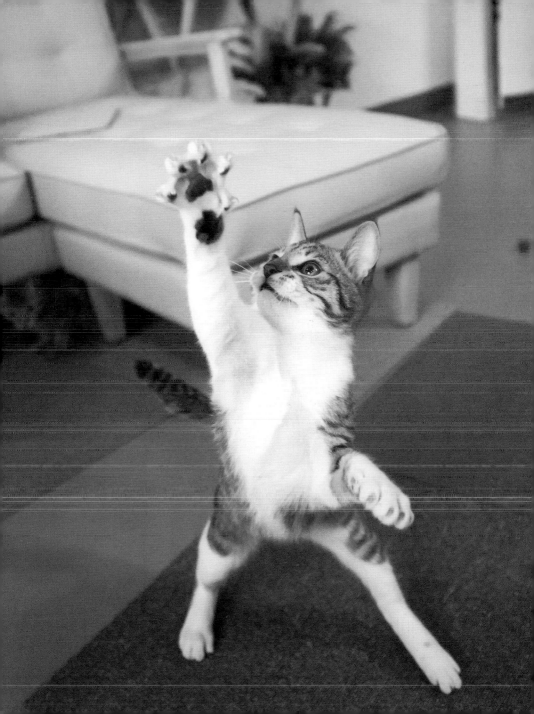

Reach Up in Triangle

Hinging from your right hip, lean your torso over your right leg, and extend your left arm up in the air.

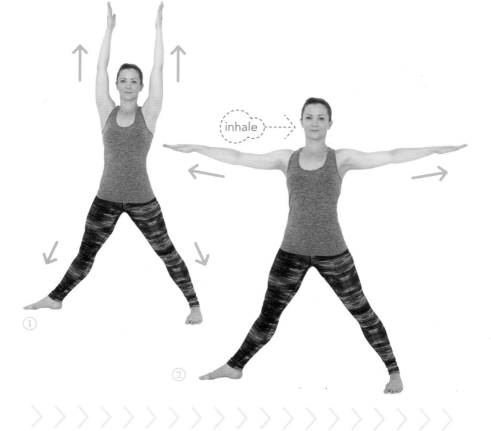

1 Stand with your legs wide apart. Turn your right toes out to 90 degrees, and turn your left toes in slightly. Lift your arms overhead, and stretch the sides of your torso as you inhale.

2 Keeping the side body and arms long, lower your arms to the height of your shoulders as you exhale. Stay here as you inhale.

Benefits:

★ ☆ ☆

■ Helps reduce tension in the back ■ Strengthens legs
■ Helps reduce stress ■ Helps improve digestion

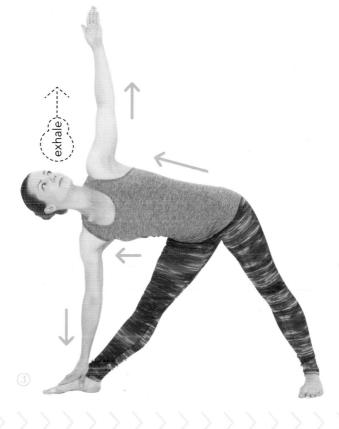

exhale

③

> >

3 As you exhale, slowly lean the right side of your torso toward the right leg, hinging from your right hip. Lower your right hand anywhere along the right leg avoiding the knee, or down to the floor if it reaches. Extend your left arm over your head. Turn your gaze toward your left hand if your neck feels comfortable. Hold for five breaths.

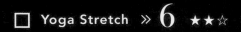

Happy Cat

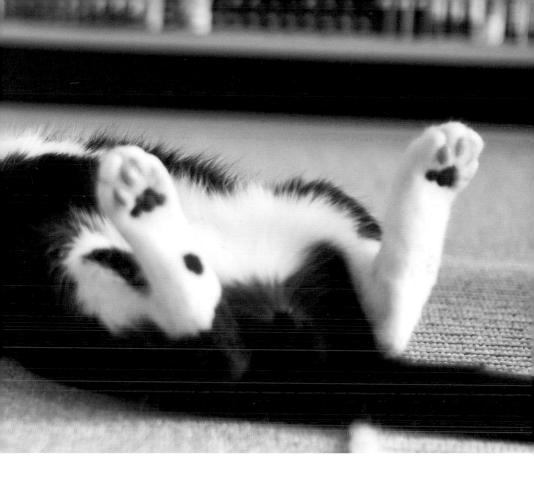

Lie down on your back, bring your knees toward your armpits, and hold onto your feet.

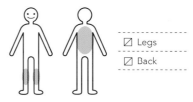

☑ Legs
☑ Back

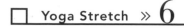

Yoga Stretch » 6

Happy Cat

Channel your inner cat by gathering your knees toward your armpits and stretching your legs long, as you roll yourself from side to side in *ananda balasana*.

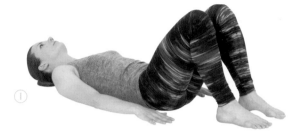

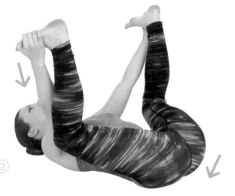

> >

1 Lie down on your back with your knees bent.

2 Bring your knees toward your armpits, and lift the soles of your feet up toward the ceiling. Hold on to your feet, ankles, or the backs of your knees.

Benefits:

- Quiets the mind ■ Help reduce stress
- May help alleviate lower back pain ■ Lessens fatigue

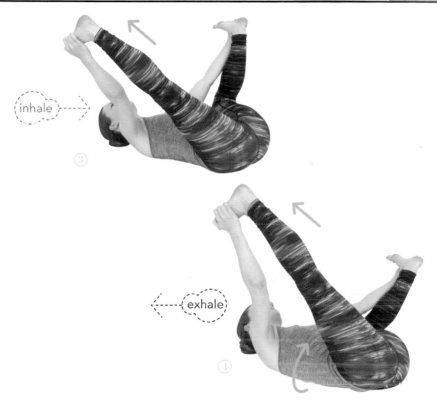

inhale ⟶

③

⟵ exhale

④

⟩ ⟩ ⟩ ⟩ ⟩ ⟩ ⟩ ⟩ ⟩ ⟩ ⟩ ⟩ ⟩ ⟩ ⟩ ⟩ ⟩

3 Start to extend your right leg diagonally toward the sky away from your left leg as you inhale. Hold for five breaths.

4 Roll to your left side, and rest your left thigh on the floor. Move your right leg farther away from the left to get a deeper inner thigh stretch. Hold for five breaths. Repeat Steps 3 and 4 on your second side.

Stick Your Tongue Out!

Open your mouth wide, and stick out your tongue.

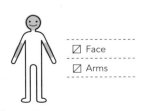

☑ Face

☑ Arms

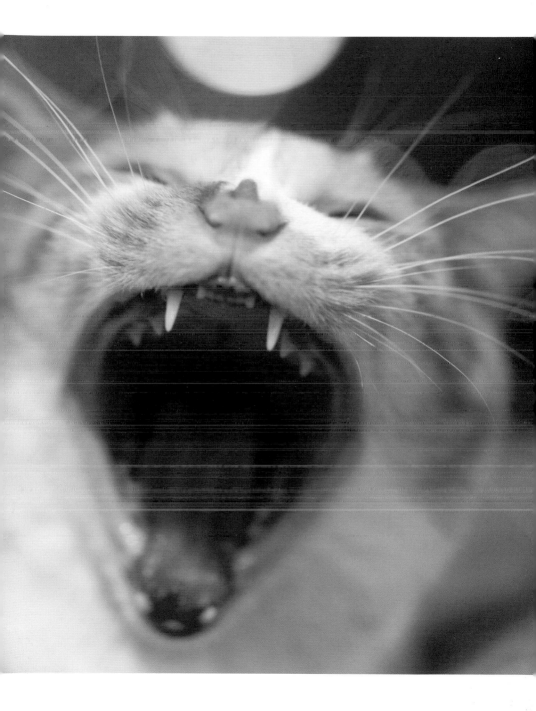

Stick Your Tongue Out!

With your mouth open wide, stick out your tongue and exhale like a cat—or even a lion!— in *simhasana*, or lion pose.

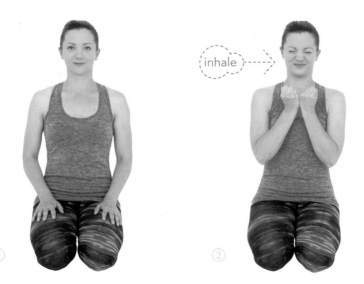

inhale ┄┄┄►

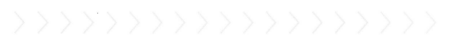

1   Sit on your heels. If this is not comfortable, you can sit cross-legged or on a chair.

2   As you inhale, close your eyes, and squeeze all your facial muscles in toward the tip of your nose. Make fists, and bring them toward your chin.

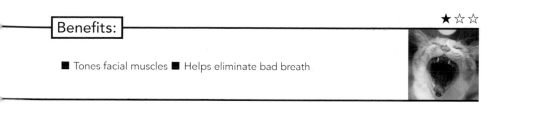

★ ☆ ☆

Benefits:

■ Tones facial muscles ■ Helps eliminate bad breath

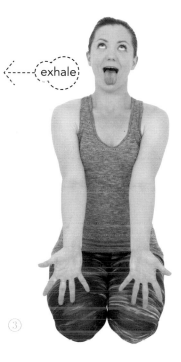

exhale

③

〉〉〉〉〉〉〉〉〉〉〉〉〉〉〉〉〉〉〉〉〉

3 As you open your mouth, stick your tongue all the way out toward the chin, roll your eyes up, exhale a big "HAAAA!" sound, and extend your arms with your palms open and fingers stretched out. Repeat Steps 2 and 3 five times.

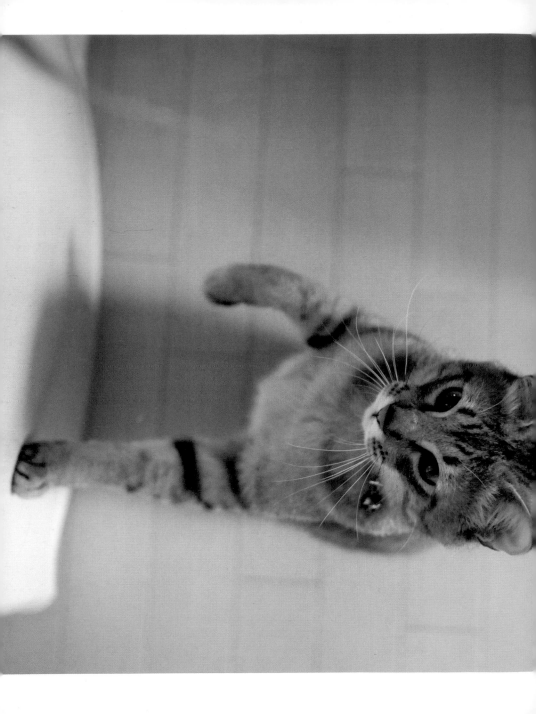

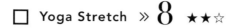

□ Yoga Stretch » 8 ★★☆

Hand at
the Wall

(with a Leg Kicking Back)

With one hand on the wall,
use your other hand to catch your foot.

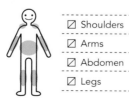

☑ Shoulders
☑ Arms
☑ Abdomen
☑ Legs

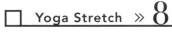

Hand at the Wall

(with a Leg Kicking Back)

Try this variation of *natarajasana*, or king dancer pose, by holding your foot to stretch the front of your thigh, optionally using the wall to help you balance.

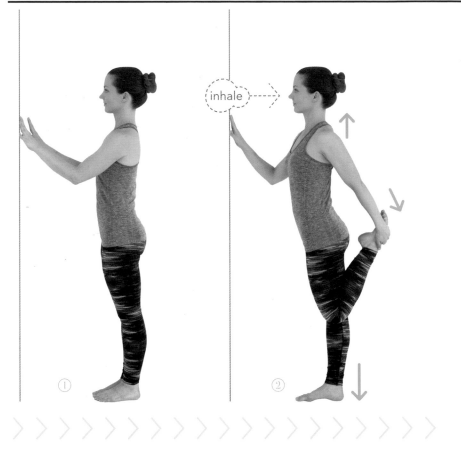

inhale

> >

1 Stand a foot or two away from the wall with your right fingertips touching the wall.

2 Keep your right hand at the wall, and as you inhale, bend your left knee to catch your foot with your left hand. Bring your knees close together.

★ ★ ☆

Benefits:

- Loosens tight shoulders ■ Tones abdominal muscles
- Improves balance ■ Strengthens legs and lower back

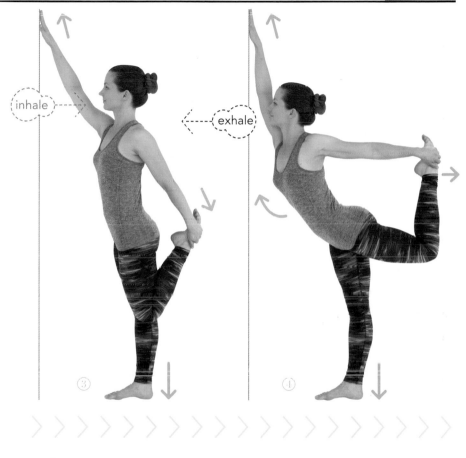

inhale

exhale

> >

3 As you inhale again, extend your right arm up toward the ceiling.

4 As you exhale, lean your torso toward the wall, and kick your foot into your hand as you move your thigh away from the wall. Hold for five breaths.

Warrior Pose

Step one foot back, and bend your front knee with your arms raised overhead.

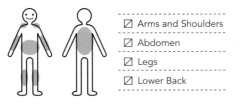

☑ Arms and Shoulders

☑ Abdomen

☑ Legs

☑ Lower Back

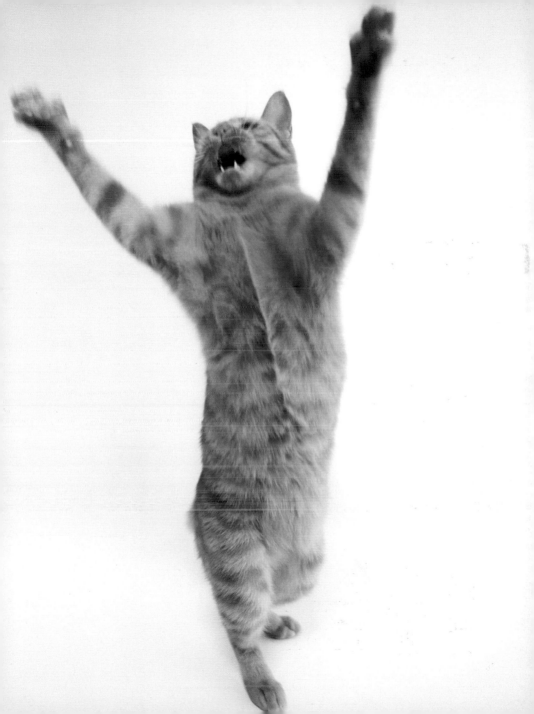

Warrior Pose

Stand strong with your back leg straight, your front leg bent, and your arms up like a warrior in *virabhadrasana 1*.

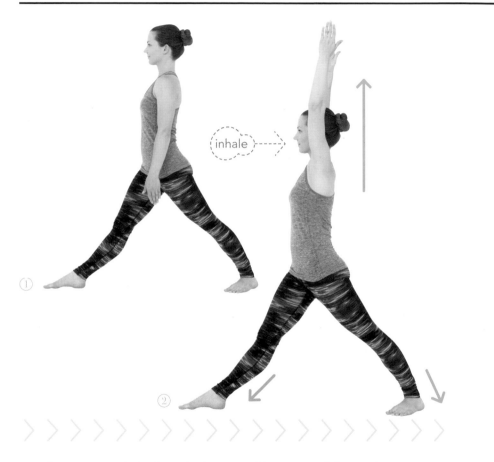

inhale

1 Step your right foot forward and your left foot back. Align your back heel to your front heel, or step your feet wider if you feel wobbly. Turn your left toes out to a 45 degree angle.

2 As you inhale, extend your arms. Keep your shoulders down with both feet firmly grounded.

Benefits:

- Loosens tight shoulders and back
- Tones buttocks ■ Strengthens legs and lower back

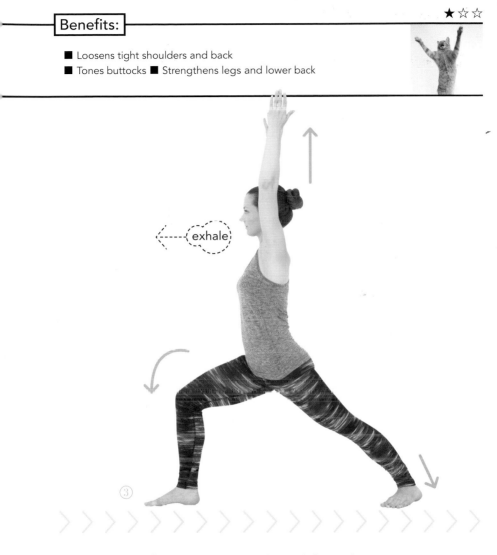

exhale

③

3 As you exhale, bend your right knee until your knee is directly above your ankle. Keep your left leg straight, and hold the pose for five breaths. Repeat on the other side.

Supine Twist

Lie down on your back with your knees bent,
and lower your legs to one side.

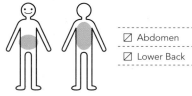

☑ Abdomen
☑ Lower Back

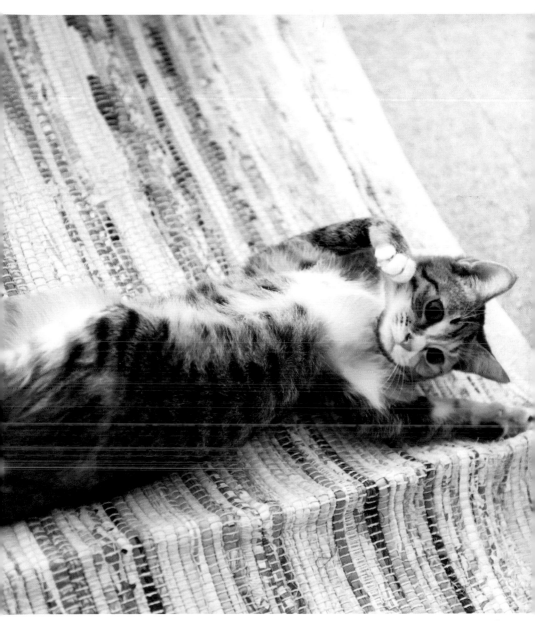

Supine Twist

Gently stretch your sides and back by twisting your torso and lowering your legs to each side in this variation of *jathara parivartanasana*.

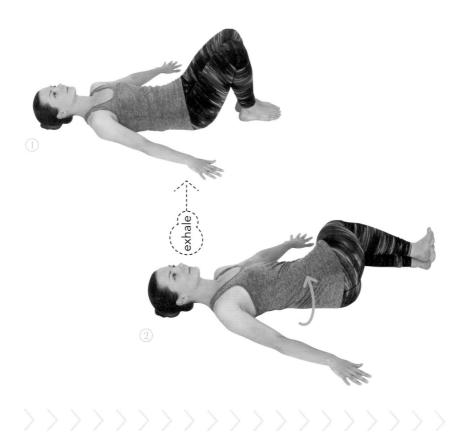

> >

1 Lie down on your back. Bring your legs together as you bend your knees and place your feet flat to the floor.

2 Move your hips slightly to your right. Then, lower your legs to the left as you exhale. Adjust your legs, so the knees are at about a 90 degree angle.

Benefits:

- Helps improve digestion ■ Helps detoxify the body
- Helps reduce stress ■ May prevent lower back pain

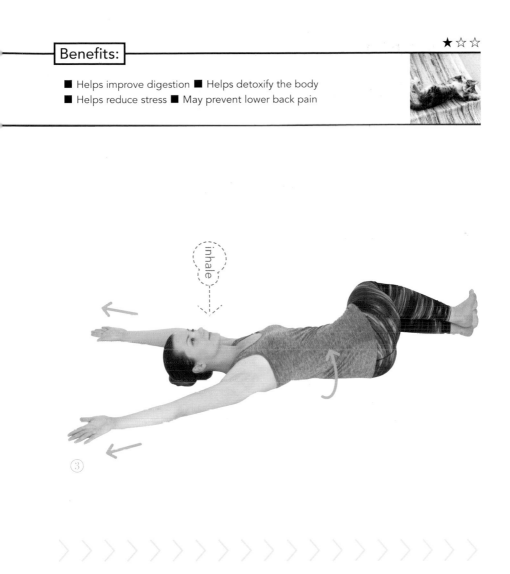

3

Reach your arms overhead, and turn
your palms to face up. Hold for five
breaths. Repeat on the other side.

Seated Twist

Sit on your heels, and turn your torso to one side.

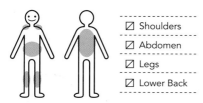

☑ Shoulders

☑ Abdomen

☑ Legs

☑ Lower Back

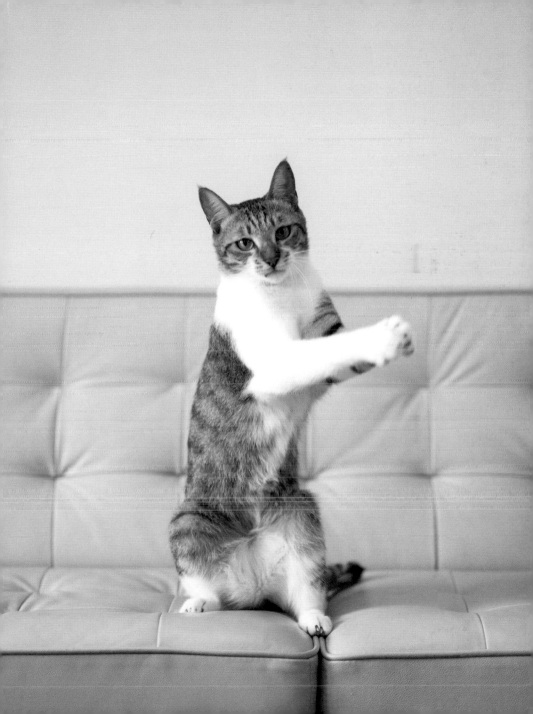

Seated Twist

To try *vajrasana*, or thunderbolt pose, sit on your heels, and turn your torso to each side, optionally bringing your hand to your waist to deepen the twist.

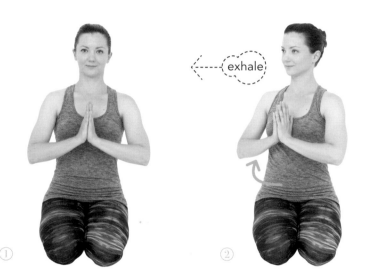

exhale

①   ②

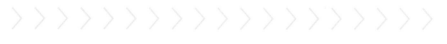

1 Sit on your heels with your hands together in front of your chest. If sitting on your heels is not comfortable, sit cross-legged or on a chair.

2 Keeping your hands together, exhale as you start to turn your torso to the right from your belly button.

Benefits:

- Loosens tight shoulders and back ■ Helps improve digestion
- Improves posture ■ Massages internal organ ■ Helps reduce stress

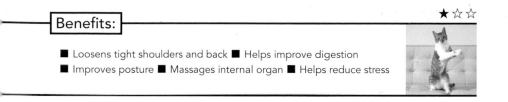

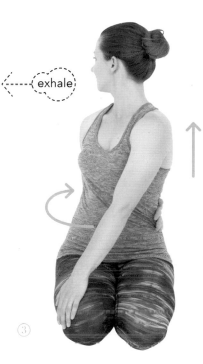

exhale

③

> >

3 Bring your left hand to your right knee and your right hand behind you. Or, place the back of your right hand behind your back to rest against the left side of your waist. Inhale to lengthen your spine, and exhale to gently twist deeper. Hold for five breaths, and repeat on the other side.

Side Stretch

Sit sideways, and lean your torso away from your hip.

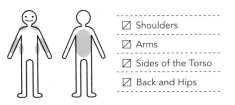

☑ Shoulders

☑ Arms

☑ Sides of the Torso

☑ Back and Hips

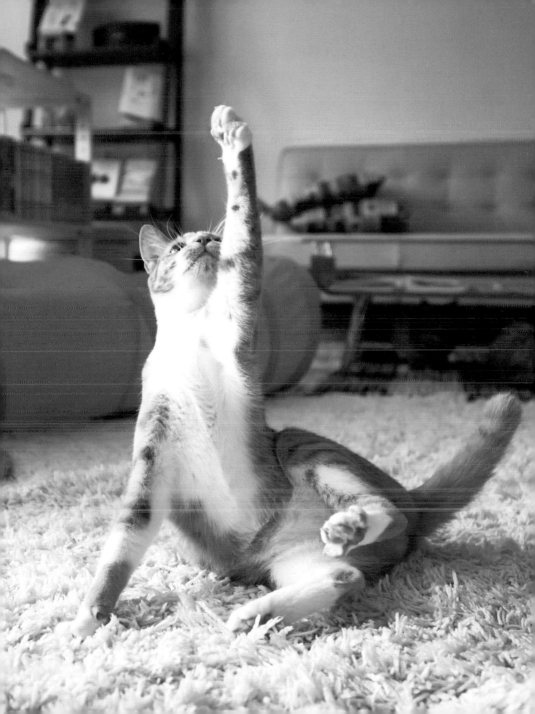

Side Stretch

Sit sideways, and bring one hand on the floor and the other overhead to feel a stretch along the side of your body.

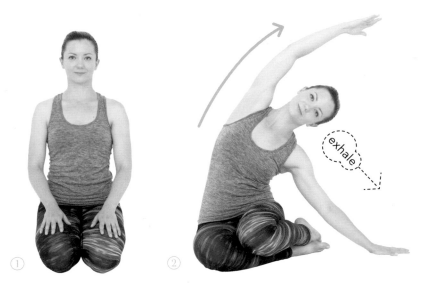

① ②

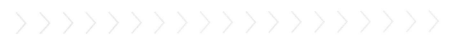

1 Sit on your heels. If it's not comfortable to sit in this position, you can sit cross-legged or on a chair.

2 Slide your hips to the right. Bring your left hand down to the floor in line with your hips. As you exhale, start to lean your torso to the left with your right arm extended alongside your ear. Hold the pose for five breaths.

Benefits:

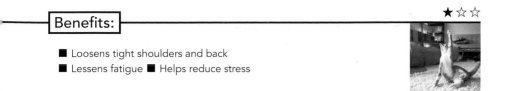

- Loosens tight shoulders and back
- Lessens fatigue ■ Helps reduce stress

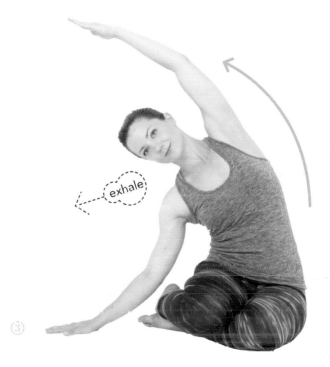

exhale

③

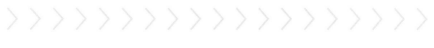

3 Bring yourself back up to the center. Repeat on the second side, and hold for five breaths.

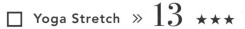

☐ Yoga Stretch » 13 ★★★

Supine Leg Stretch

Lie down on your back and lift one leg toward ceiling for a nice, juicy stretch.

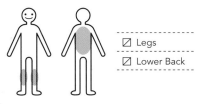

☑ Legs
☑ Lower Back

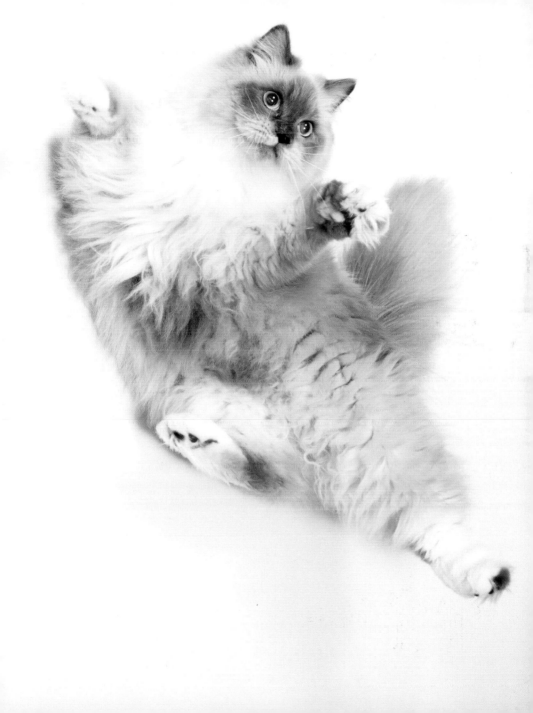

Supine Leg Stretch

Lie on your back, and come into *supta padangusthasana*, or reclining hand-to-big-toe pose, by holding onto your toe, lifting your leg, and opening it out to the side.

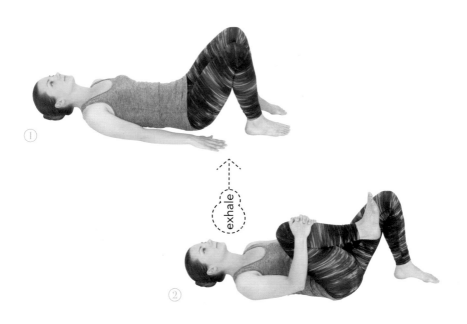

> > > > > > > > > > > > > > > > > > > >

1 Lie down on your back with your knees bent and your feet flat on the floor.

2 As you exhale, bring your right knee into your chest.

Benefits:

- Helps prevent and relieve lower back pain
- Improves circulation in the legs ■ Helps relieve constipation

inhale

exhale

③

④

> >

3 Take hold of your right big toe with your first two fingers and thumb wrapped around your big toe, or hold onto the back of your knee or thigh. Extend your leg up toward the ceiling as you inhale. You can stay here for five breaths.

4 Ground your left hip down with your left palm, and open your right leg to the side. Hold for five breaths.

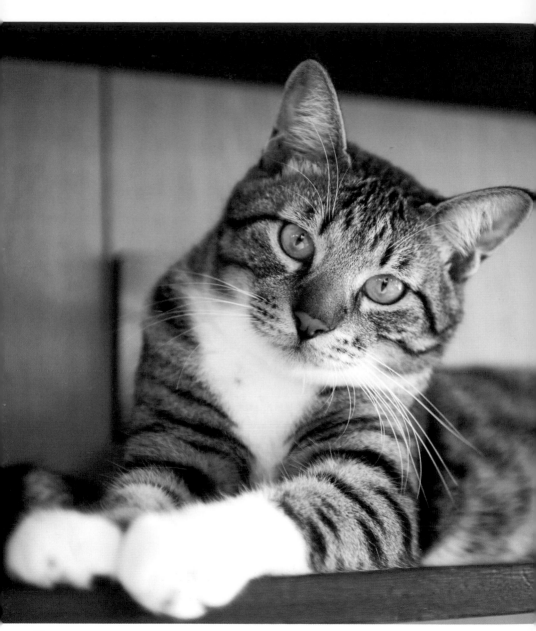

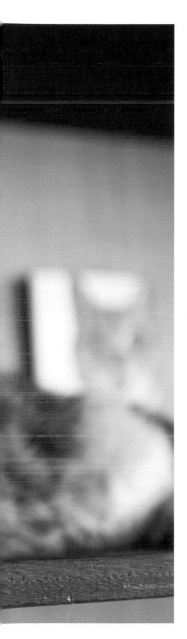

Sphinx Pose

Lie down on your belly,
and prop yourself up on your forearms.

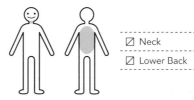

☑ Neck

☑ Lower Back

Sphinx Pose

Transform yourself into the famous Great Sphinx by lying on your belly, stretching your legs long with your toes back, placing your forearms on the floor, and lifting your torso.

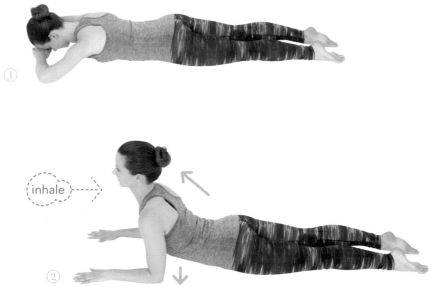

①

inhale

②

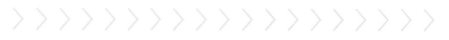

1 Lie down on your belly, and rest your forehead on your stacked hands.

2 Lift your head, neck, and chest to prop yourself up on your forearms. Your forearms should be parallel to each other, and your elbows should be directly under your shoulders.

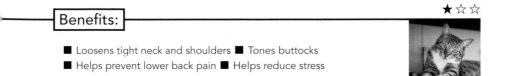

Benefits:

- Loosens tight neck and shoulders ■ Tones buttocks
- Helps prevent lower back pain ■ Helps reduce stress

★ ☆ ☆

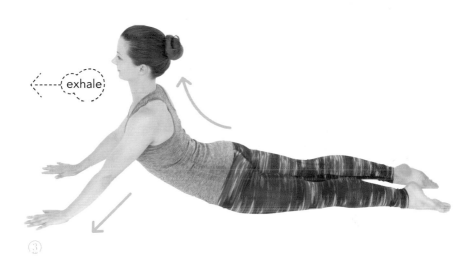

exhale

> > > > > > > > > > > > > > > > > > > >

3 If your lower back feels fine, press your hands into the ground to lift your elbows and straighten your arms. Allow your shoulders to relax away from your ears, and hold the pose for five breaths.

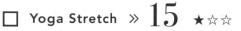

□ **Yoga Stretch** » 15 ★☆☆

True
Cat Pose

Come to all fours, and arch and round your back.

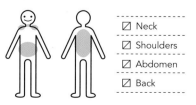

☑ Neck

☑ Shoulders

☑ Abdomen

☑ Back

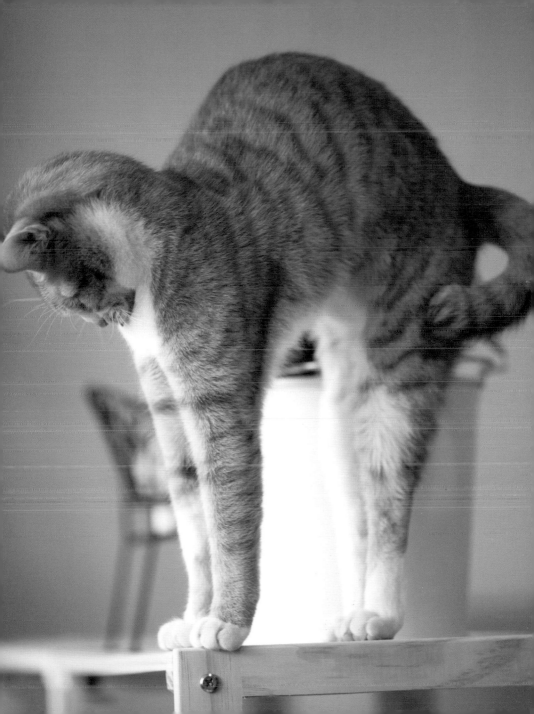

True Cat Pose

Stretch the front and back of your body by rounding and arching your spine—in the style of one of your cat's favorite moves!—appropriately named *marjaryasana*, or cat pose.

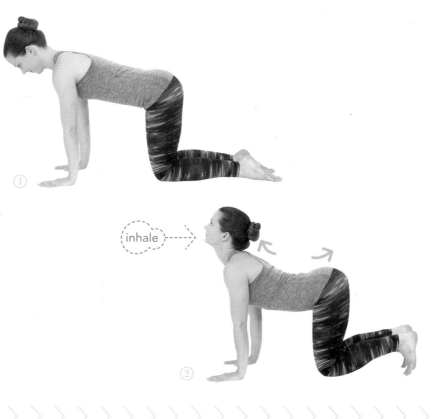

inhale

>>>>>>>>>>>>>>>>>>>>>>>

1 Come to all fours with your wrists directly under your shoulders and your knees directly under your hips.

2 As you inhale, arch your back by lifting your tailbone, looking forward and up, and tucking your toes.

Benefits:

- Loosens tight neck and shoulders ■ Helps prevent lower back pain
- Helps reduce stress ■ Massages internal organs

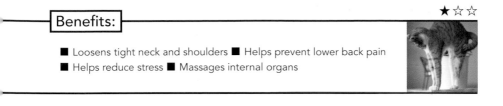

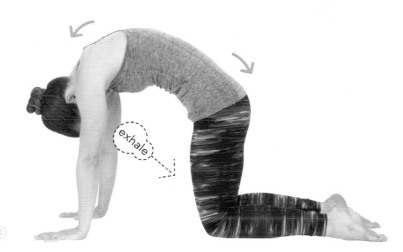

exhale

③

> > > > > > > > > > > > > > > > > > >

3 As you exhale, round your spine by tucking your tailbone , nodding your chin into your chest, and untucking your toes. Repeat Steps 2 and 3 five times.

Balance with Arms Crossed

Cross your legs, cross your arms, and balance.

☑ Neck and Shoulders

☑ Arms and Legs

☑ Back

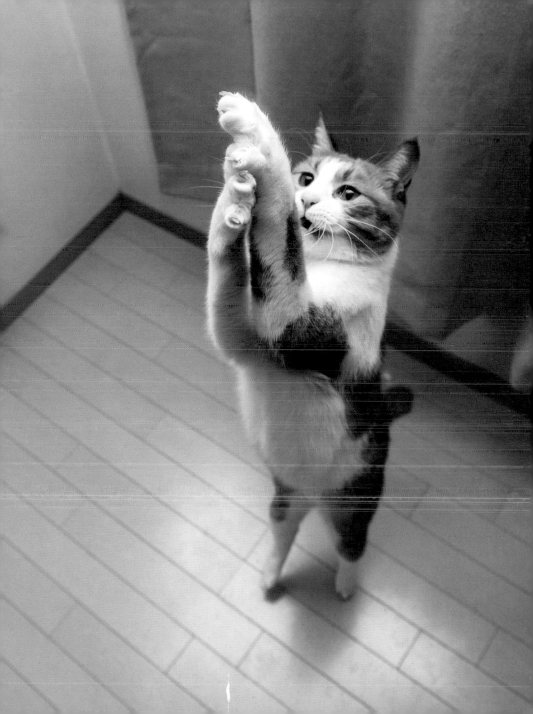

Balance with Arms Crossed

On one foot, cross your legs and arms, and optionally fold forward into *garudasana*, or eagle pose.

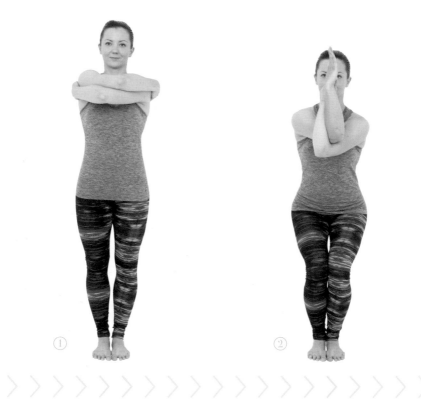

① ②

1 Stand with your feet together.

2 Then, you have three choices. Cross your right arm over the left, and hug your shoulders. Or, bring the back of your left fingers to touch the back of your right hand. Or finally, double cross your forearms, so the left fingers touch the right palm. No matter which variation you choose, bend your knees.

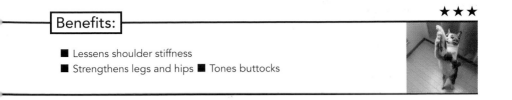

Benefits:

- Lessens shoulder stiffness
- Strengthens legs and hips ■ Tones buttocks

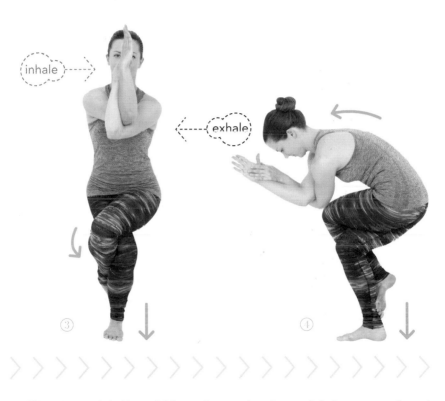

inhale ┄┄>

<┄┄ exhale

③   ④

> > > > > > > > > > > > > > > > > > > >

3 As you inhale, lift your left leg, and cross your left knee over the right. Optionally, bring the back of your left foot behind the right calf.

4 As you exhale, lean your torso forward, bringing your elbows toward your knees. Hold the pose for five breaths. Repeat on the other side.

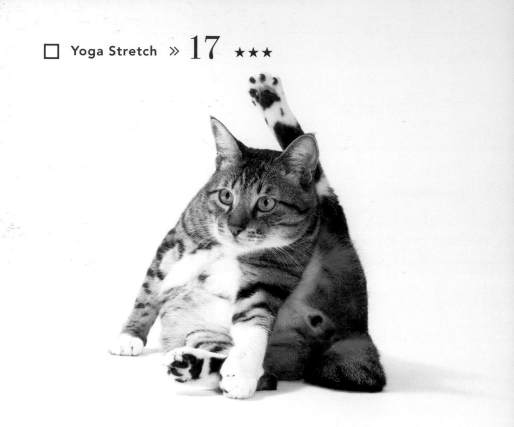

Hoist a Leg!

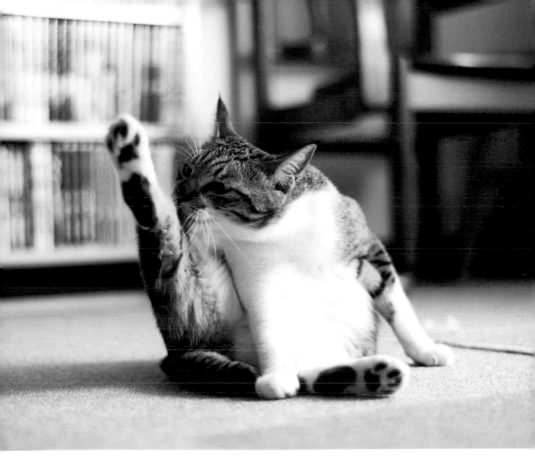

From a cross-legged seat, lift and stretch your leg over your shoulder.

☑ Side Body

☑ Legs

Hoist a Leg!

Lift a leg over your shoulder, and stretch it diagonally toward the ceiling into *parivrtta surya yantrasana*, or compass pose.

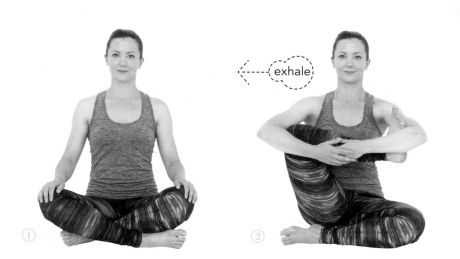

exhale

1 Sit with your right leg in front of the left.

2 As you inhale, bring your right shin toward your chest, and exhale.

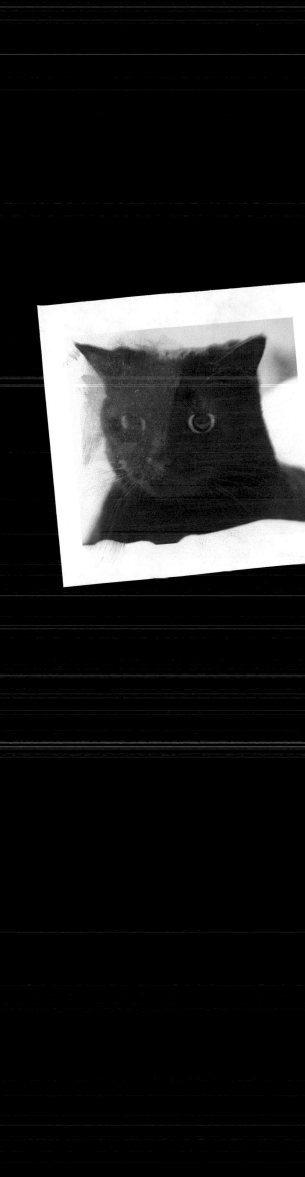

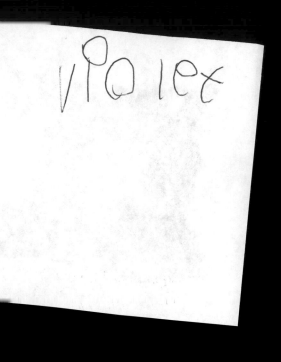

violet

Benefits:

- Helps reduce stress and raise your spirits
- Helps improve digestion

★ ★ ★

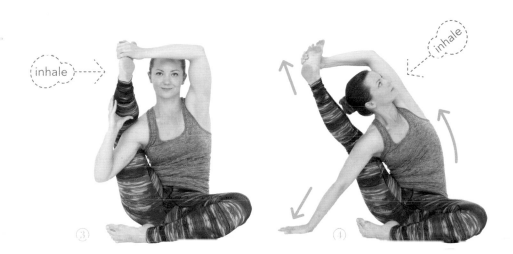

inhale

inhale

③

④

> > > > > > > > > > > > > > > > > > > >

3 As you inhale again, hoist your right leg behind your shoulder by holding your right foot with your left hand and supporting your calf with your right hand.

4 Continuing to hold the top of your right foot with your left hand, extend your right arm to the ground on the right side. On an inhalation, start to extend your right leg as much as you can without straining. Turn your gaze toward your left upper arm if it feels comfortable in your neck, and hold the pose for five breaths. Repeat on the other side.

73

Shoulders Up + Down

Lie down flat on your back,
and alternate lifting your arms and shoulders.

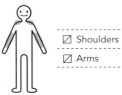

☑ Shoulders

☑ Arms

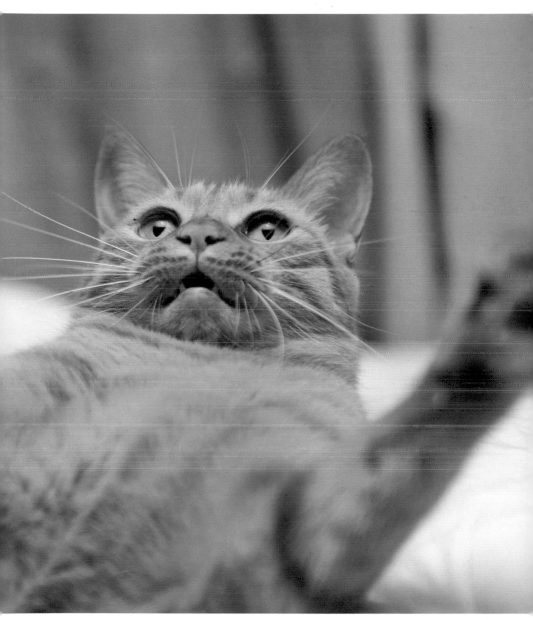

Shoulders Up + Down

From the floor, lift one arm and even shoulder off the ground, while you bend the elbow on your other arm, and then switch.

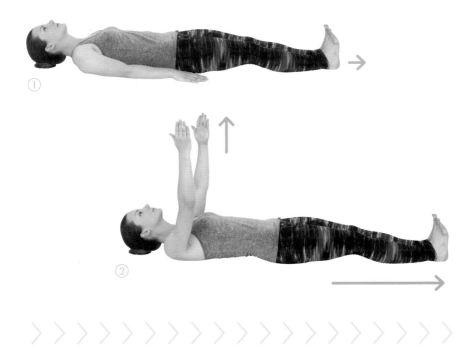

①

②

>>>>>>>>>>>>>>>>>>>>>

1 Lie down on your back with your legs together, and press your heels forward.

2 Extend your arms straight up toward the ceiling with your palms facing one another.

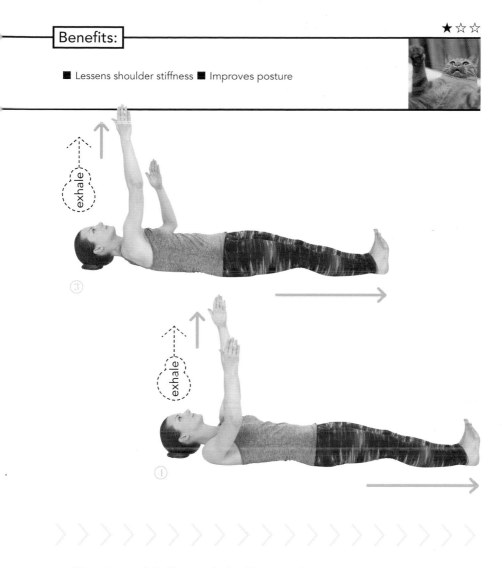

3 As you exhale, lift your right shoulder off the ground as you bend your left elbow slightly. Inhale to return your right shoulder down.

4 As you exhale, switch sides, and lift your left shoulder up as you bend your right elbow slightly. Inhale to return your left shoulder down. Repeat this for five left-and-right sets.

☐ **Yoga Stretch** » 19 ★☆☆

Twist on a Lazy Day

With your legs wide and knees bent, twist.

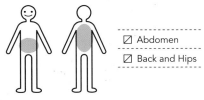

☑ Abdomen

☑ Back and Hips

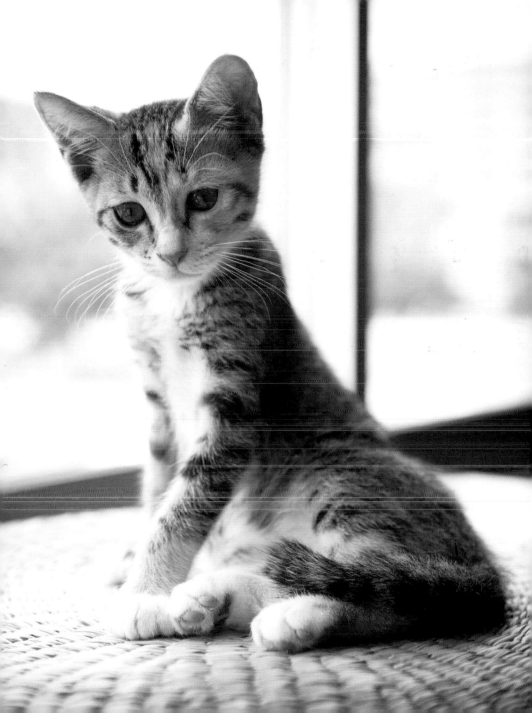

Twist on a Lazy Day

The perfect stretch for a day when you are feeling tired or run down, this gentle torso twist starts from a seated position with your feet flat, knees bent, and arms behind you.

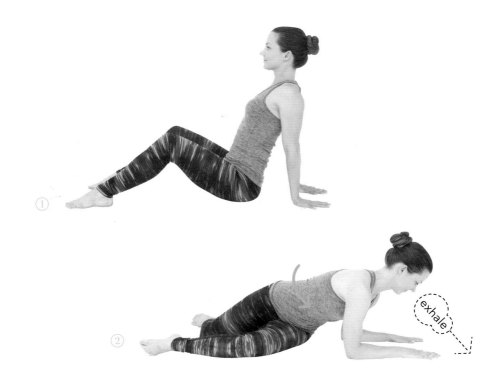

exhale

1 Sit with your knees bent and feet wider than your hips. Lean back and prop yourself up with your hands.

2 As you exhale, lower your legs all the way to the left, as you twist your torso in the same direction. Lower both forearms down behind you.

- Massages internal organs ■ Helps prevent lower back issues
- Helps reduce stress ■ Helps detoxify the body

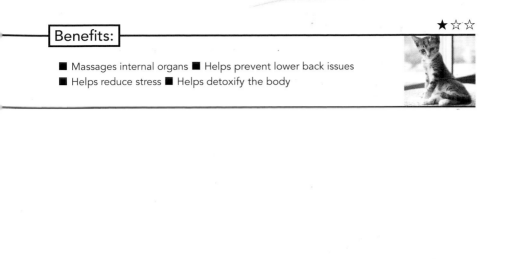

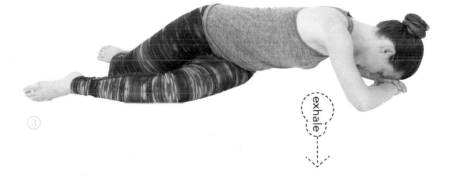

exhale

③

3 As you exhale, lower your forehead on your stacked hands. Stay there for five breaths, and then repeat the stretch on the other side.

Legs
Wide + Fold

Sit with your legs wide, and fold forward.

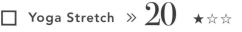

☑ Legs

☑ Back and Hips

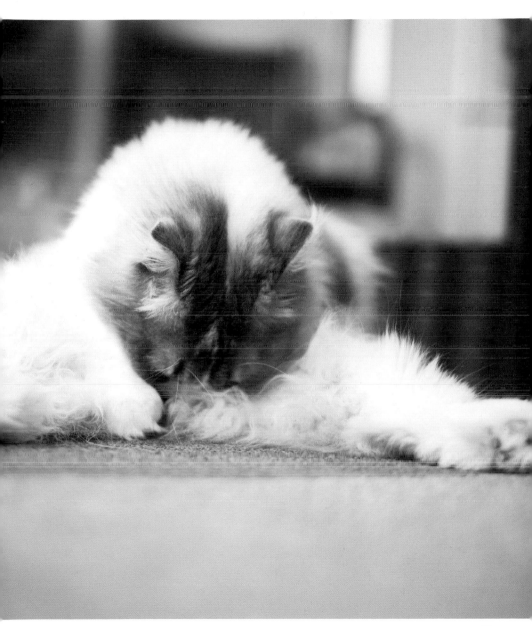

Legs Wide + Fold

Try one of the most popular poses, *upavstha konasana*, to stretch the backs of your legs, your inner thighs, and your entire back, being sure to lengthen your spine before folding forward.

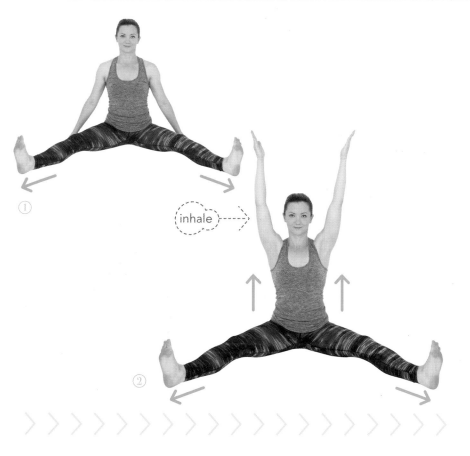

inhale

1 Sit with your legs wide. Press your heels away from you.

2 As you inhale, lift your arms overhead. Make sure you lengthen your spine first to get a deeper stretch.

Benefits:

■ Lessens fatigue ■ May help alleviate headaches
■ Helps reduce stress ■ Helps alleviate lower back pain

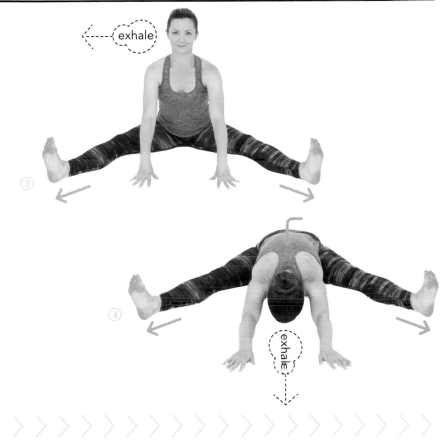

exhale

③

exhale

④

> >

3 As you exhale, place your hands in front of you.

4 Inhale to re-lengthen the spine, and as your exhale hinge from your hips to fold forward a little deeper, stretching your arms forward. Stay for five breaths.

Lie on Your Side Stretch

Lie down on your side, and separate your legs.

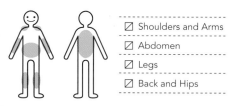

☑ Shoulders and Arms

☑ Abdomen

☑ Legs

☑ Back and Hips

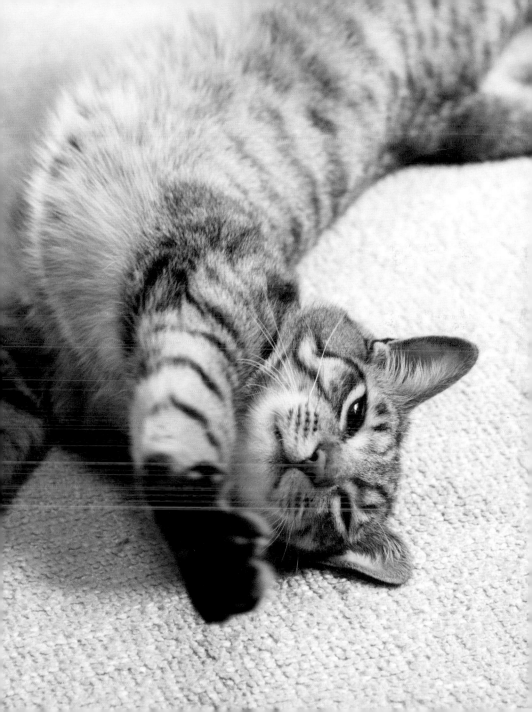

☐ Yoga Stretch » 21

Lie on Your Side Stretch

To take after your cat and enjoy a stretch for your whole body, lie on your side, separate your legs with one ahead of you and one behind, and arch your back.

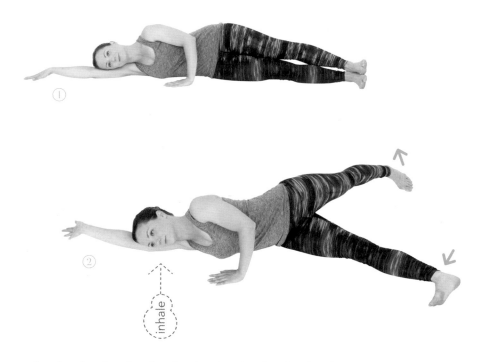

inhale

1 Lie on the right side of your body. Rest your head on your right arm with your left hand on the ground in front of your torso for an easier time balancing.

2 As you inhale, move your right leg forward and your left leg back, separating your legs as wide as you can.

★ ☆ ☆

Benefits:

■ Loosens tight shoulders and back ■ Strengthens core

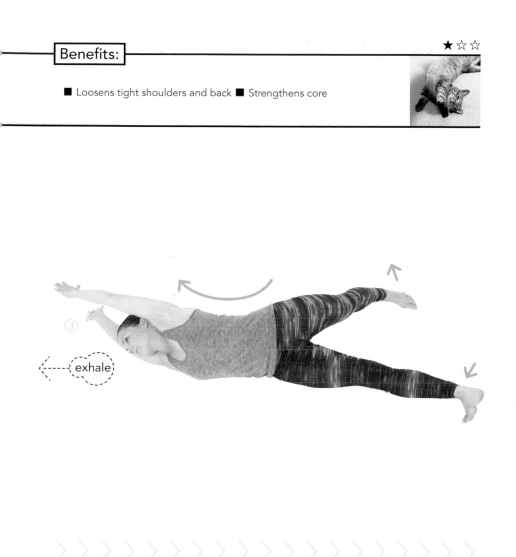

exhale

3 As you exhale, arch your torso back and bring your left arm overhead. Hold for five breaths, and then switch sides.

Go Upside-Down

Come to all fours with your feet at the wall,
lift your knees, and start to walk up the wall.

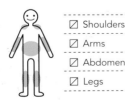

☑ Shoulders

☑ Arms

☑ Abdomen

☑ Legs

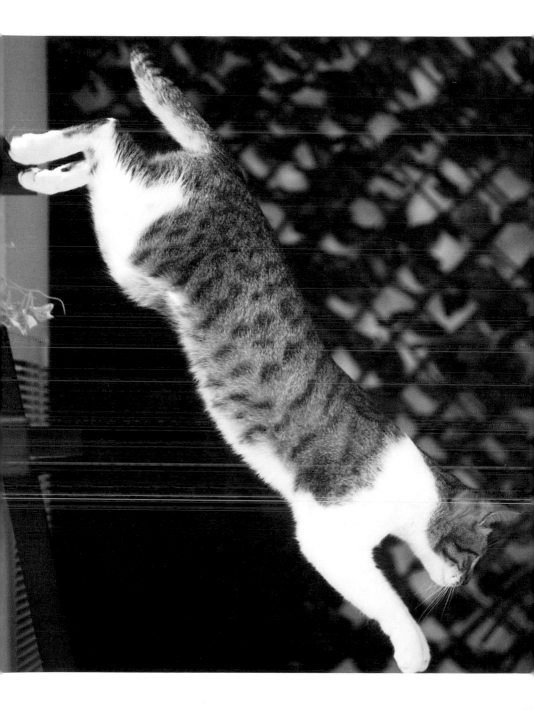

Go Upside-Down

Come to all fours with your feet at the wall, straighten your legs, and start to lift one leg and then the other to go upside-down in this variation of *adho mukha vrksasana*, or downward facing tree pose.

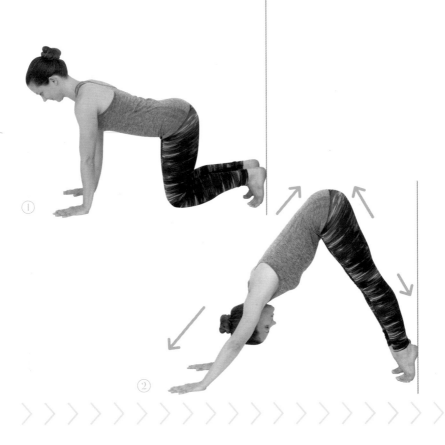

1 Bring your knees and hands to the floor with the soles of your feet touching the wall.

2 Lift your knees and hips into an inverted "V" shape.

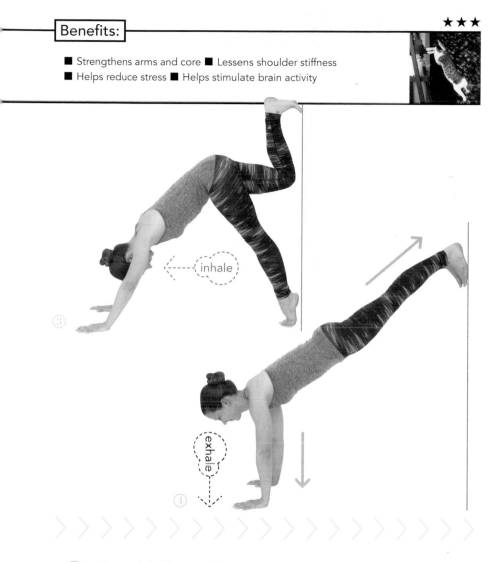

inhale

exhale

3   As you inhale, lift one leg, and push your toes against the wall to lift your other leg.

4   Walk your feet up the wall to begin straightening your legs. Optionally, walk your hands closer to the wall as you keep walking your feet toward the ceiling. Stay for five breaths, but make sure you save enough strength to walk your hands forward to safely come out of the shape.

Sit on Your Heels

Lean back while sitting on your heels to stretch your thighs.

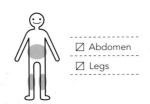

☑ Abdomen

☑ Legs

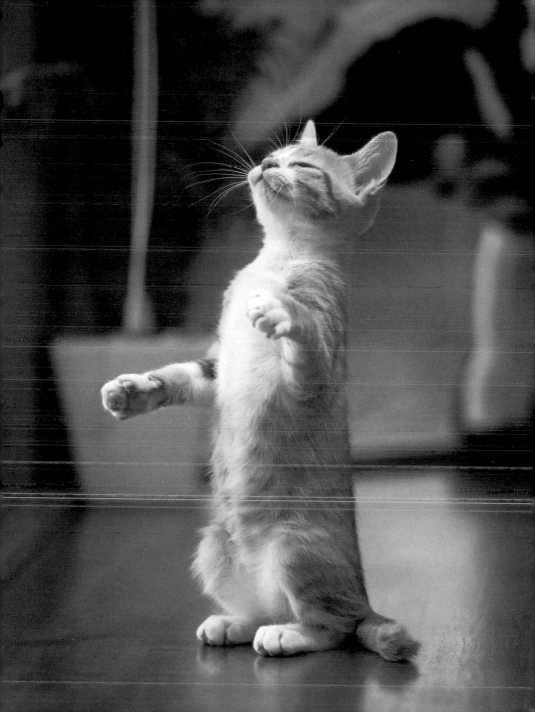

Sit on Your Heels

The pose is called *ustrasana*, or camel pose, and you can try it by sitting on your heels and leaning back to stretch your thighs and abdomen.

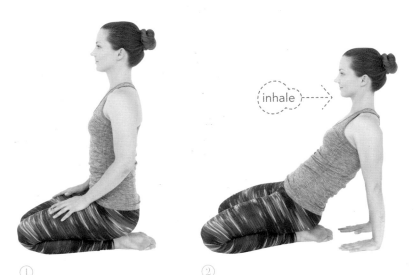

inhale

①   ②

>>>>>>>>>>>>>>>>>>>>>>>>>>>>>>

1 Sit on your heels with your feet together. Lengthen your spine, and keep your eyes on the horizon.

2 Open your knees slightly, and as you inhale, bring your hands behind you, turning your fingers toward your hips.

- Helps improve digestion ■ Helps relieve constipation
- Helps reduce mild depression

★ ☆ ☆

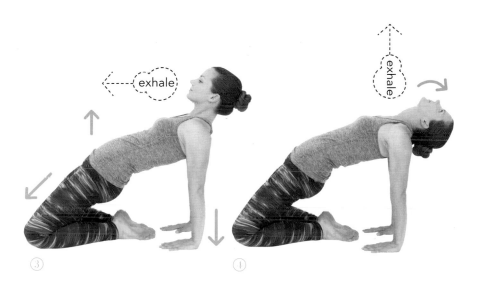

exhale

exhale

③ ④

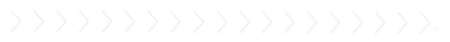

3 As you exhale, lift your hips up.

4 If it feels comfortable for your neck, drop your head back. Hold the pose for five breaths.

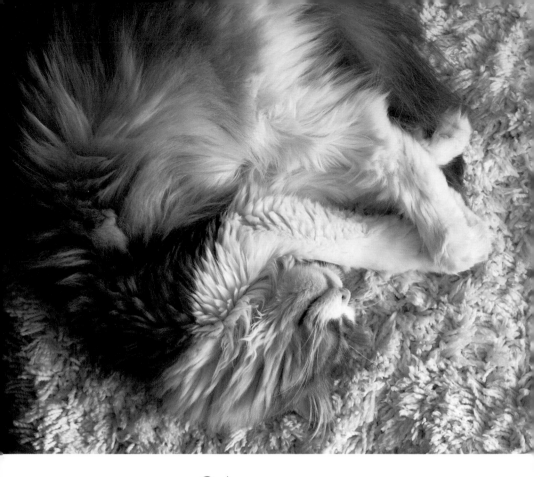

□ Yoga Stretch » 24 ★☆☆

Turn into a Ball

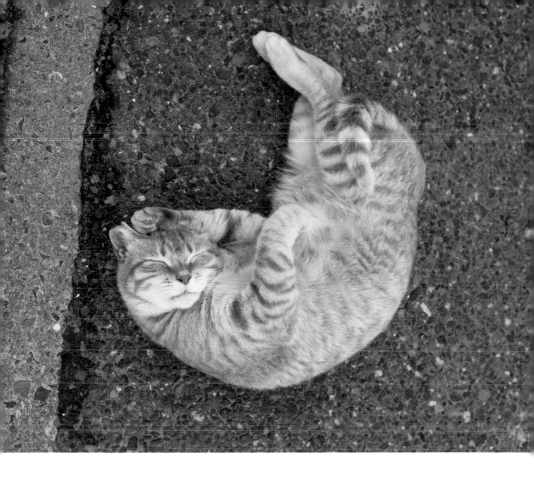

Lie on your back, and hug your knees into your chest.

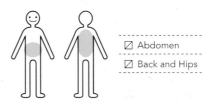

☑ Abdomen
☑ Back and Hips

Turn into a Ball

Bring your knees and head toward one another to make yourself into a ball. The pose is called *apanasana*, wind-relieving pose.

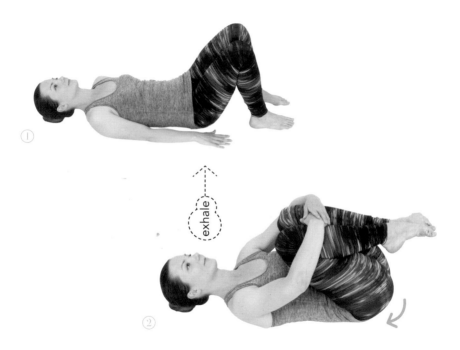

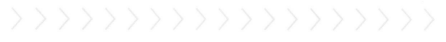

1 Lie down on your back with your knees bent.

2 As you exhale, bring your knees toward your chest.

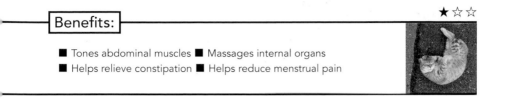

- Tones abdominal muscles ■ Massages internal organs
- Helps relieve constipation ■ Helps reduce menstrual pain

exhale ┄┄┄>

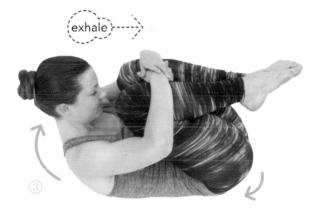

③

3

As you exhale, lift your head, and bring
your forehead toward your knees. Hold
for five breaths.

Lie on Your Belly Stretch

Lift your arms and legs, one at a time or all at once.

☑ Arms

☑ Abdomen

☑ Legs

☑ Back and Hips

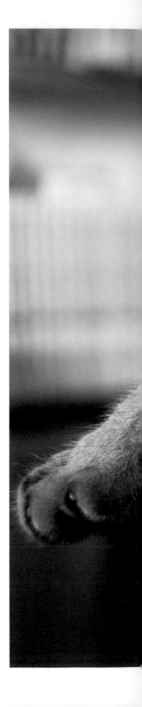

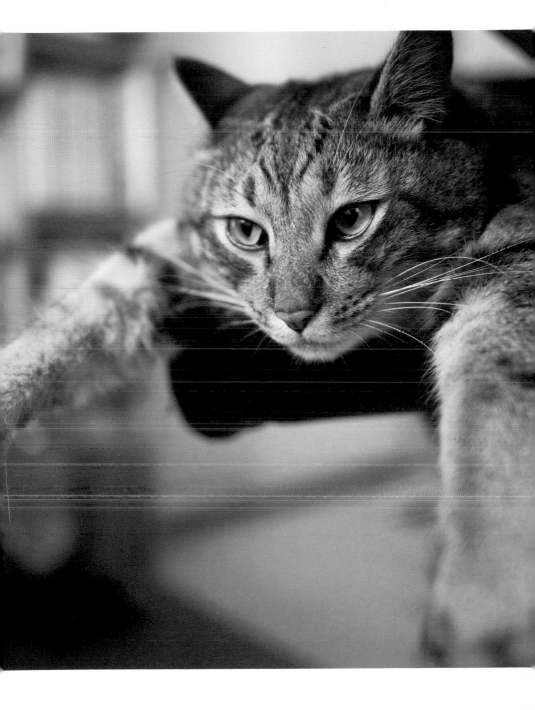

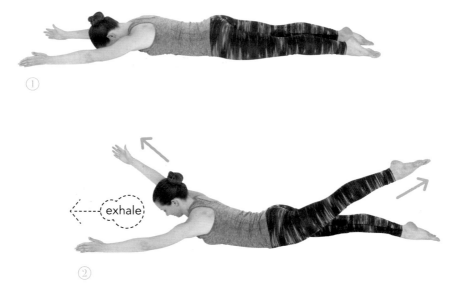

Lie on Your Belly Stretch

Facing the floor, extend your arms overhead, lift your opposite arm and leg, switch to the other side, and then lift everything at once!

exhale

1 From your belly, place your feet hip-distance apart. Extend your arms overhead with your palms facing one another and your forehead resting on the floor.

2 As you exhale, lift your right arm, your left leg, and your torso. Keep your limbs stretched long.

★ ☆ ☆

Benefits:

■ Loosens tight shoulders and back ■ Strengthens back muscles
■ Helps improve digestion ■ Helps alleviate lower back pain

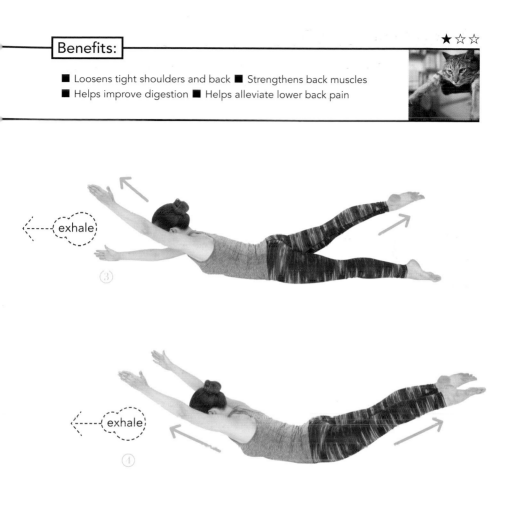

exhale

③

exhale

④

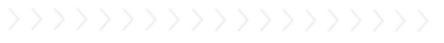

3 As you inhale, lower yourself down. Exhale to switch sides, stretching your opposite arm and leg away from one another.

4 Inhale to come down from your second side. Optionally, exhale to lift both arms and legs at the same time. Repeat Steps 2 to 4 five times.

Stick Your Butt Out

Bend your knees, lower your hips behind you, and reach your arms up overhead.

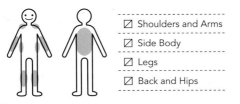

☑ Shoulders and Arms

☑ Side Body

☑ Legs

☑ Back and Hips

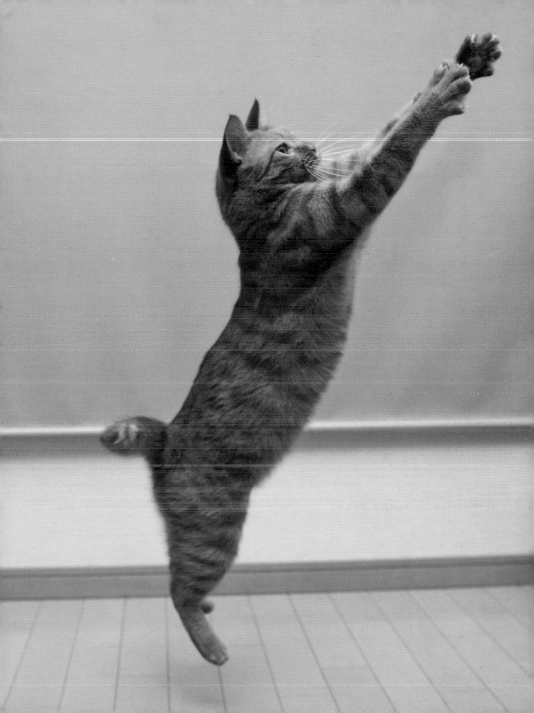

Stick Your Butt Out

The pose is called *utkatasana*, or chair pose, and you can try it simply by bending your knees and sitting down...onto an imaginary chair!

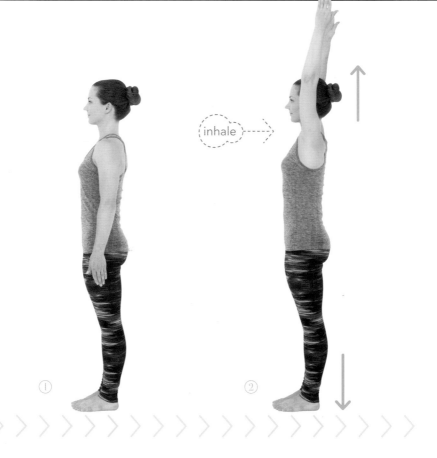

inhale ╌╌╌►

①

②

1 Stand with your feet together, and lengthen your spine.

2 As you inhale, lift your arms overhead or out in a wide "V" shape.

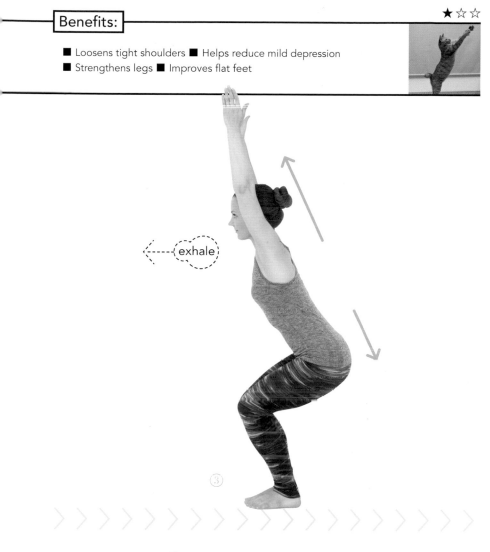

exhale

③

3 As you exhale, bend your knees, and stick your butt out and down behind you as you lean your torso forward. Keep your arms reaching alongside your ears or out wide. Hold for five breaths.

Down Dog

From bent knees and arms extended, rise to all fours,
and then straighten up and back to down dog.

☑ Shoulders

☑ Arms

☑ Legs

☑ Back and Hips

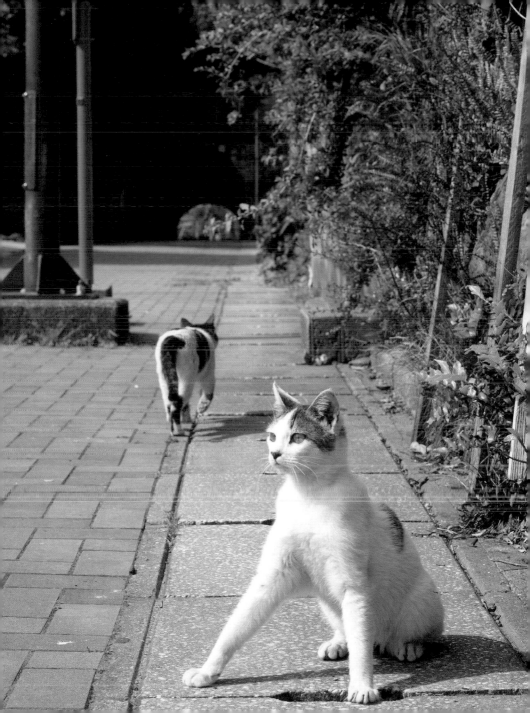

Down Dog

This sequence takes you from child's pose with your arms extended to all fours to down dog with your hips lifted high.

exhale

①

inhale

②

1 Sit on your heels with your knees wide, and fold forward with your forehead on the floor. Reach your arms long overhead, palms facing the ground in child's pose.

2 As you inhale, rise to knees and hands.

Benefits:

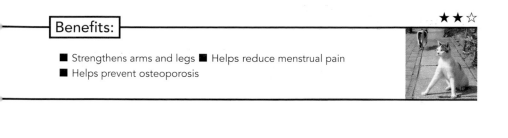

- Strengthens arms and legs ■ Helps reduce menstrual pain
- Helps prevent osteoporosis

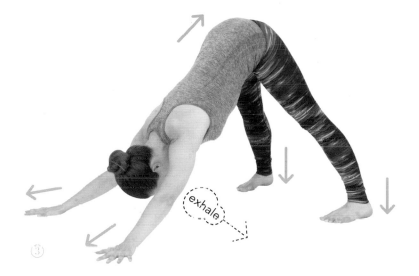

exhale

> >

3 As you exhale, lift your hips up, and begin
extending your legs. Press your palms flat to the
floor, and move your hips away from your hands
to help lengthen the spine. Keep your gaze
toward your feet. Stay for five breaths.

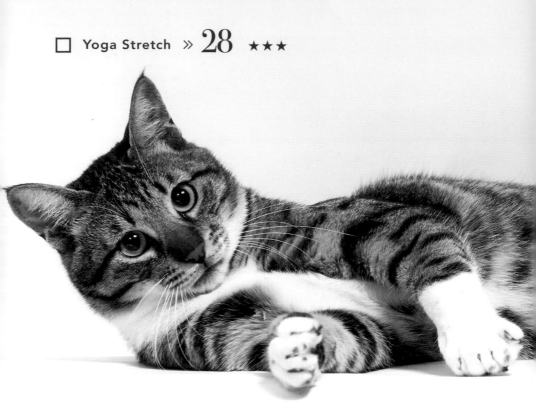

Side-Lying
Leg Lift

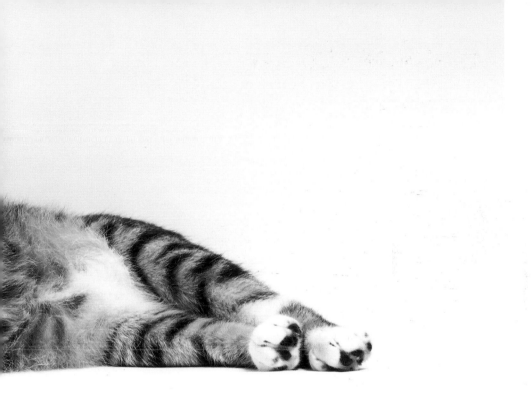

Lie on your side, and lift your top leg toward the ceiling.

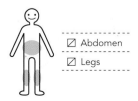

☑ Abdomen

☑ Legs

Side-Lying Leg Lift

Lie down on your side with your top leg lifted toward the ceiling in *anantasana*, a pose that helps promote both flexibility and balance.

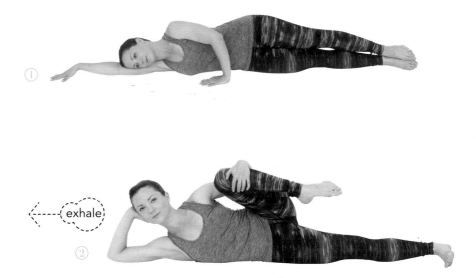

exhale

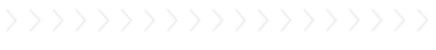

1 Lie down on your right side with your legs stacked together. Rest your head on your right arm and place your left palm in front of you for help balancing.

2 As you exhale, bring your left knee toward your left armpit. Hold the knee with your left hand.

- Helps improve digestion ■ Tones buttocks ■ Improves balance
- Helps alleviate lower back pain ■ Strengthens core

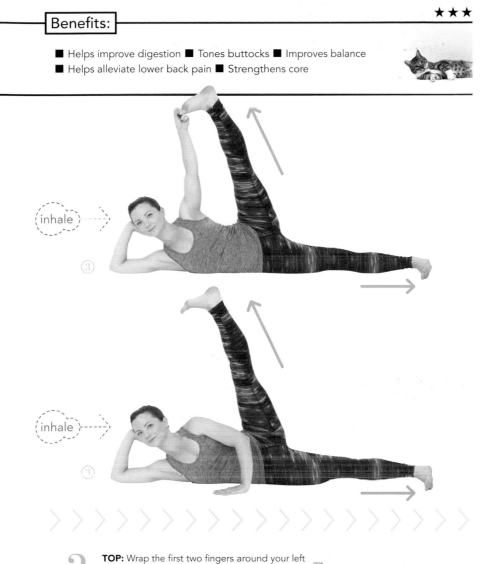

inhale

③

inhale

③

3 **TOP:** Wrap the first two fingers around your left big toe, and lift your leg toward the ceiling.

BOTTOM: Or, keep your hand in front of you, and lift your leg.

Hold either version of the pose for five breaths, and then repeat on the other side.

Top of Your Head Down

Gently backbend with your legs long
and the top of your head resting on the floor.

☑ Neck
☑ Back

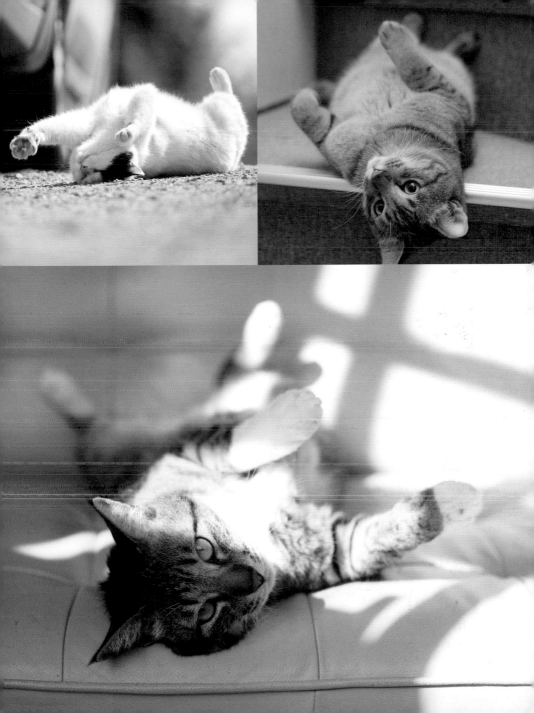

Top of Your Head Down

With your legs extended, slowly lean back, and bring the top of your head down into *matsyasana*, or fish pose.

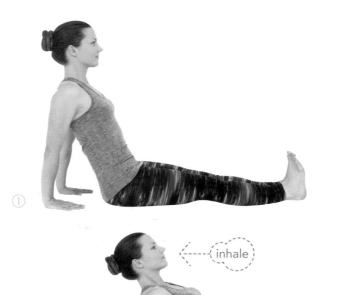

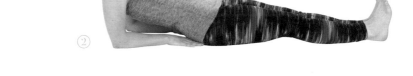

1 Sit and extend your legs in front of you. Lean back with your hands behind you, turning your fingers to point toward your hips.

2 As you inhale, slowly lower yourself down to your forearms.

Benefits:

- Loosens tight shoulders and back
- Helps improve respiration ■ Helps reduce mild depression
- Helps alleviate lower back pain ■ Lessens fatigue

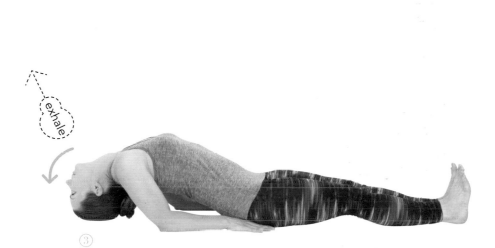

exhale

③

> >

3 As you exhale, move your forearms and hands toward your feet, as you slowly allow the top of your head to reach toward or rest on the floor. Hold the pose for five breaths.

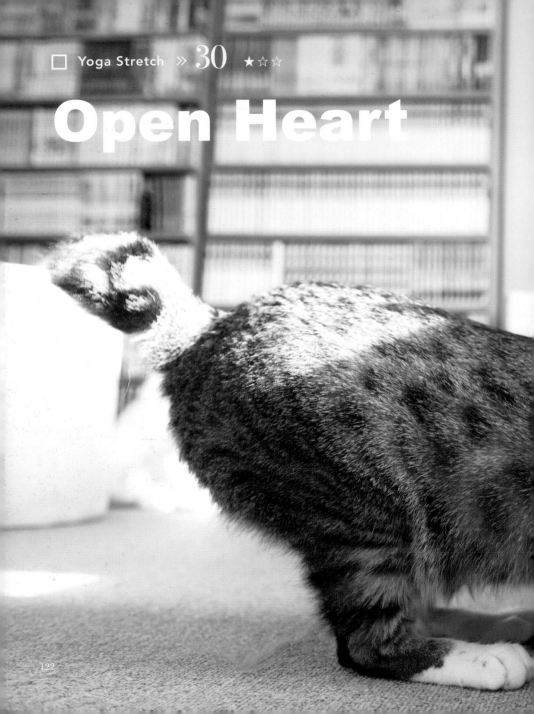

Open Heart

Stretch your arms forward
with your knees and forehead on the floor.

☑ Shoulders

☑ Arms

☑ Back

Open Heart

From all fours, stretch your arms forward, and lower your forehead down into *anahatasana*, or puppy dog pose.

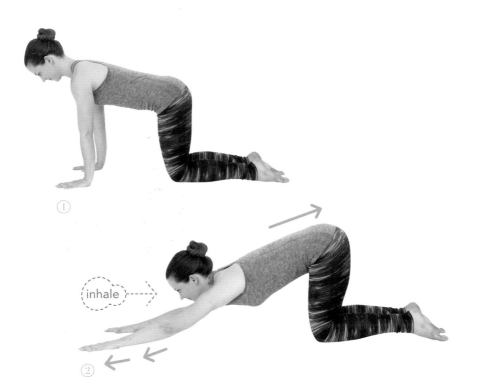

inhale ⤏

① ②

1 Come to all fours with your hips directly over your knees—and not in front of or behind them. Lengthen your spine, including the back of your neck.

2 As you inhale, start to extend your arms forward but keep your hips over your knees.

Benefits:

■ Loosens tight shoulders ■ Improves posture

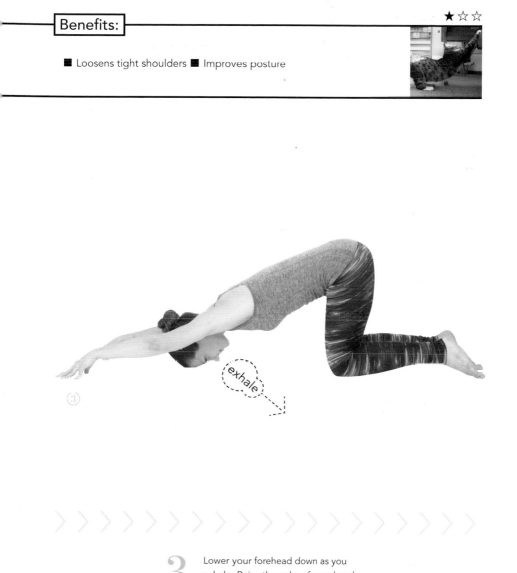

exhale

③

3 Lower your forehead down as you exhale. Raise the palm of your hands, but leave your fingertips on the ground. Hold for five breaths.

□ **Yoga Stretch** » 31 ★☆☆

Relax + Rest

Lie down on your back,
and relax with your eyes closed.

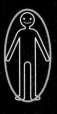

☑ Entire Body

☑ Mind

Relax + Rest

Lie down on your back with your arms slightly away from your body and your feet wider than your hips in *savasana*, or corpse pose—yes, this is a real yoga pose!

Benefits:	■ Relaxes body and mind ■ Helps reduce stress ■ Lessens fatigue ■ Lowers blood pressure ■ May help alleviate headaches

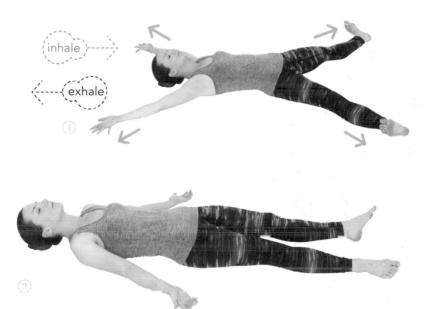

inhale

exhale

$\large{1}$ Lie down on your back with your legs at least as wide as your hips and your arms reaching overhead so that your whole body is shaped like the letter "X." Hold for five breaths.

$\large{2}$ Bring your arms by your side, palms facing up, and bring your feet slightly wider than your hips, with your feet falling open. Close your eyes, and stay for 5–10 minutes.

Yoga with Cats: 31 Yoga Stretches Inspired by Cats

Published in 2017 by:
NIPPAN IPS Co., Ltd.
1-3-4, Yushima
Bunkyo-ku, Tokyo, 113-0034

ISBN 978-4-86505-099-8

NEKOYOGA
©Transworld Japan Inc. 2016
Original Japanese edition is published by Transworld Japan, Tokyo, Japan.

Editorial Supervisor & Translator: Masako Miyakawa

English Language Editor: Hilary Hudgins
http://hilaryhudginspoetry.com

Cat Model Photographer: Akimasa Harada
https://www.flickr.com/photos/rampx/

Human Model Photographer: Mami Yamada
http://www.mamiyamada.jp/

Model: Karin Ahlin
http://www.karinahlin.com/

Shot in cooperation with Be Fluent NYC
http://www.befluentnyc.com

Design: Yoko Komatsu
Commissioning Editor: Aya Nihei
Editorial Director: Fuyuko Kita
Publisher of Japanese Edition: Hiroshi Sano

Printed in China